Carol H.
please return

Captain LeVrier Believes In Miracles

Kathryn Kuhlman

Captain LeVrier Believes In Miracles

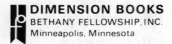
DIMENSION BOOKS
BETHANY FELLOWSHIP, INC.
Minneapolis, Minnesota

ISBN 0-87123-077-1

DIMENSION BOOKS
are published by Bethany Fellowship, Inc.
6820 Auto Club Road, Minneapolis, Minnesota 55438

Printed in the United States of America

Captain John LeVrier

John LeVrier is a Captain in the Houston Police Department, Houston, Texas. A native Texan, he is also an active deacon in the First Baptist Church of Houston.

Table of Contents

Table of Contents

1. The Shock Hits

I have been a policeman since I was twenty-one years old. I started with the Houston Police Department back in 1936 and worked my way up to the rank of Captain of the Accident Division. In all those years I had never been sick. But in December, 1968, when I went in for a physical examination, things changed.

I had known Dr. Bill Robbins since he had been an intern and I was a rookie cop. He used to ride with me in my prowl car when I first started on the force. Following what I thought was a routine physical exam in his office in the St. Joseph's Professional Building, Dr. Robbins pulled off his rubber gloves and sat on the end of the table. He shook his head. "I don't like what I find, John," he said. "I want you to see a specialist."

I glanced at him as I tucked my shirt in my pants and buckled my gun belt around my waist. "A specialist? What for? My back hurts some, but what cop's back. . . ."

He wasn't listening. "I'm going to send you right on up to see Dr. McDonald, a urologist in this same building."

I knew better than to argue and two hours later, following an even more thorough examination, I was listening to another physician, Dr. Newton McDonald. He minced no words. "How soon can you go into the hospital, Captain?"

"Hospital?" There was just a tinge of fear in my voice.

"I don't like what I find," he said deliberately. "Your prostate gland should be about the size of a hickory nut, but it's the size of a lemon. The only way I can tell what is wrong is run a biopsy. We can't wait. You ought to be in the hospital no later than tomorrow morning."

I went straight home. After supper Sara Ann put the three children to bed. John was only five, Andrew seven, and Elizabeth nine. Then I broke the news.

She listened quietly. We'd had a happy life together. "Don't put it off, John," she said evenly. "We have too much to live for."

I looked at her, leaning up against the edge of the kitchen counter, so young, so pretty. I thought of our three beautiful children already in bed. She was right, I did have a lot to live for.

Three evenings later, after extensive hospital examinations (including the biopsy), I sat propped up in my bed at the hospital, eating dinner. The door to my room opened. It was Dr. McDonald and one of the doctors on the hospital staff. They closed the door and then pulled up chairs beside my bed. I knew busy doctors didn't have time to chat socially and I felt my pulse begin to throb in my throat.

Dr. McDonald didn't leave me guess-

13

ing long. "Captain, I'm afraid we have some distressing news." He paused. The words were hard to utter. I waited, trying to keep my eyes focused on his lips. "You have cancer."

I saw his lips move and form the word, but my ears refused to register the sound. Over and over I could see the word on his lips. Cancer. Cancer. Just like that. One day I'm as strong as an ox, a veteran of 33 years on the police force. The next day I have cancer.

It seemed like an eternity before I could respond. "Well, which way do we go? I guess you'll have to take it out."

"It's not that simple," he said, clearing his throat. "It's malignant and too far advanced for us to handle it here. We're referring you to the doctors at the M.D. Anderson Tumor Institute. They're known all over the world for their research in cancer treatment. If anyone can help you, they can. But it doesn't look good, Captain, and we would be lying if we held out any hope for the future."

2. Cobalt Barrage

Both doctors were sympathetic. I could tell they were moved, but they knew I was a veteran police officer and would demand the facts. They gave them to me as frankly, yet as gently, as they could. Then they left.

I sat looking at the cold food on my tray. Everything seemed lifeless. The coffee, the half-eaten swiss steak, the apple sauce. I pushed it away and swung my legs over the side of the bed. Cancer. No hope.

Walking to the window I stood looking out over the city of Houston, a city which

I knew better than the back of my hand. It was cancerous too, filled with crime and disease like any big city. For a third of a century I had been working trying to stop the spread of that cancer, but it seemed like an endless task. The sun was just setting and its dying rays caught the spires of the church steeples rising above the rooftops. I'd never noticed, but Houston seemed to be filled with churches.

I was a member of one of them, the First Baptist Church. In fact, I was an active deacon in the church, although my personal faith didn't amount to much. Some of my friends at the department used to kid me and say I was the same kind of Baptist that Harry Truman said he was, the Bourbon-drinking, poker-playing, cussing type. Even though I had heard my pastor preach some mighty sermons on salvation, I'd never had any victory in my personal life. I was a deacon by virtue of my position in the community, rather than because of my spirituality. Now here I was, face to face with death, groping for something to stand on. But as I put my feet down into the water there was no bottom. I felt as if I were sinking.

I looked down from the ninth floor. It would be easy just to go on through the window. I'd seen men die of cancer, their bodies eaten out by the disease. How much easier it would be simply to end it now. But something Sara had said stuck with me. "We have too much to live for. . . ."

I walked back to the bed and sat on the edge, staring into the gray-black dusk that seemed to be closing in on me. How would I tell her, and the kids, that I was going to die?

The next day the doctors from the M.D. Anderson Institute came in. There were more tests. Dr. Delclose, the doctor in charge of my case, really got honest with me. "All I can tell you is you had better be prepared to see an awful lot of doctors," he said.

"How long do I have?" I said.

"I can't give you any hope," he said frankly. "Maybe a year, maybe a year and a half. The cancer is very extensive in your entire lower abdomen. The only way we can treat it is with massive doses

17

of radiation, which means we'll have to kill a lot of healthy tissue at the same time. However, if we are to prolong your life at all, we must get started."

I signed a release and they started cobalt treatment the same day.

I believed in prayer. We used to pray for the sick every Wednesday night at the First Baptist Church. But we prefaced our prayer for healing with the words, "If it's Your will, heal. . . ." That is the way I had been taught. I knew nothing of praying with authority—the kind of authority that Jesus and the apostles had. I believed that God was certainly able to heal people, but I just assumed that He wasn't in the miracle-performing business today.

Thus, when I went into radiation, my body shaved and marked off with a blue pencil like a side of beef ready for the butcher's cleaver, the only prayer I knew to say was, "Lord, let this machine do what it was designed to do."

Now that's not a bad prayer, for the machine was designed to kill cancer cells. Of course the doctors were trying to keep the radiation from affecting the rest of my organs, so I was marked off to the millimeter. The cancer was in the prostate area and had to be treated from all angles, so the huge cobalt machine circled the table, the radiation penetrating my body from every side.

The treatments lasted for six weeks, one a day. I was released from the hospital and allowed to go back to work, coming in each morning to receive the cobalt.

3. The Cancer Spreads

Four months passed after I had been diagnosed. Easter was approaching and Sara mentioned that it looked like it would be happier than Christmas. Maybe the cobalt had done its job, or even better, maybe the doctors had made a mistake. Then, just 120 days after the first diagnosis, the pain hit.

It was a Friday noon. I had promised to meet Sara at the little restaurant where we often met for lunch. She had already arrived. I grinned, laid my policeman's cap on the window sill, and slipped into the booth beside her. As I sat down I felt like I had been stabbed with a white hot dagger. The pain surged through my right hip in excruciating spasms. I was unable to speak and just looked at Sara in mute agony. She grabbed my arm.

"John," she gasped, "what is it?"

The pain slowly subsided, leaving me so weak I could hardly talk. I tried to tell her; then, like the tide moving in over the salt flats, it returned. It was like fire in my bones. My face beaded with perspiration and I pulled at my collar to loosen my tie. The waitress, who had come to take our order, sensed something was wrong. "Captain Le-Vrier," she said with concern, "are you all right?"

"I'll make it," I finally said. "I've just had a sudden pain."

But we decided not to eat. Instead we went straight to the hospital and Dr. Del-close immediately set up more X-rays. As they were preparing me I put my hand on my right hip and could feel the indentation. It was about the size of a silver dollar and felt like a hole under the skin. The X-rays showed it up for what it was: the cancer had eaten a hole all the way through my hip. Only the outer skin was covering the cavity.

"I'm sorry, Captain," the doctor said with resignation. "The cancer is spreading as expected."

Then in measured tones he concluded: "We'll start the cobalt again and do everything we can to make your time as painless as possible."

The daily trips to the hospital began all over again.

Sara tried to be calm. She had worked in the Police Department before our marriage and had been exposed to death many times. But this was different. I didn't know it at the time, but the doctors had told her that I probably had no more than six months to live.

I kept on working, although I was growing weaker and weaker. It was hard to determine whether it was the cancer or cobalt. One afternoon Sara picked me up from work and said, "John, I've been thinking. I've been out of circulation a long time. What would you say if I went back to work?"

"You've got a job," I kidded. "You

23

just take care of those three children and I'll earn the bread around this house. I've still got a lot of mileage left in me."

"Still the tough cop, aren't you?" she said. "Well, I'm tough too. I'm going to enroll in business college."

It began to dawn on me what she was doing. She was getting things in order. It was time for me to do the same thing. But before I could, a new development took place—surgery.

"It's the only way to keep you alive," the woman surgeon said. "This type of cancer feeds on hormones. We are going to have to redirect the hormone trend in your body through surgery. If we don't do this, you are really going out fast."

24

4. "I Believe in Miracles"

I agreed to the surgery but within another 120 days the cancer reappeared on the surface. This time in my spine.

I first noticed it on a Saturday afternoon in June. Sara had taken the children to a Vacation Bible School picnic and I was home, trying to set out a little potted plant in the flower bed. By now I was so weak I could hardly bend over, but I thought the exercise would help. I had dug a small hole in the ground and bent over to pick up the potted plant when the pain, like a million volts of lightning, surged through my lower back. I fell forward into the dirt.

I never dreamed such pain could exist. No one was around to help me so I dragged myself, partially on my hands and knees, partially on my stomach, up the steps and into the house. Then, for the first time, I let myself go. Lying on the floor in that empty house, I wept and moaned uncontrollably. I had been holding back because of Sara and the children, but this afternoon, with the house empty, I lay there crying and moaning until the pain finally subsided.

There followed another series of cobalt treatments with more hopeless looks from the doctors. I had received the death sentence.

Cancer takes you apart from the inside, and I wasn't the only one in my family dying. We received word that my two sisters' husbands, who also lived in Houston, had cancer. The disease spread rapidly and they were both dead in months. Both of these men were in their early fifties, my own age bracket. I realized I was next. It was time to finish getting things in order.

I had always wanted a big, old car. I splurged and bought a three-year-old Cadillac. As the summer ended we packed the family into the car and set out on what I thought was to be my last vacation. I wanted to make it a good one for the children. Years before I had traveled through the Pacific northwest and I wanted Sara and the children to see that part of the world which had meant so much to me: the Columbia River Drive, Mt. Hood, the coast of Oregon, Lake Louise, Yellowstone and the Rocky Mountains. The children didn't know, but Sara and I both believed it would be our last summer together as a family.

I returned to Houston and tried to patch up loose ends. But when life is frayed beyond splicing, it's impossible to pick up the strings. All you can do is let them dangle and wait for the end.

One Saturday morning, in the early fall, I walked into the den and turned on the TV. Our pastor at the First Baptist Church, John Bisango, had a program called "Higher Ground." John had come to Houston from Oklahoma where his church had been recognized as the most evangelistic church in the Southern Baptist Convention. What had happened in Oklahoma was beginning to happen in Houston as this dynamic young pastor began to turn that huge church right side up. I was thrilled with his ministry.

Too weak to get up, I sat slumped in the chair as the program ended. "I believe in miracles," a woman's voice said. I glanced up. I wasn't impressed, very few Baptists are impressed about a woman preacher. But as the program progressed and this woman, Kathryn Kuhlman, talked of wonderful healing miracles, something inside me clicked. "Can this be for real?" I wondered.

The show closed and the credits were flashed on the screen. Suddenly I saw a familiar name: Dick Ross, producer.

I knew Dick. I had known him since 1952 when he was in Houston working with Billy Graham producing "Oiltown, USA." In fact, I had played a bit roll in that movie and as a result had become a good friend of Billy Graham and his team, remaining in charge of his security detail whenever he came to Houston. Now, here was Dick Ross's name, only this time associated with this woman preacher who talked about healing miracles.

I had kept in contact with Dick across the years. When I would have to go to California on police work, I always looked him up. I had visited in his home, even sat in on his Sunday school class at the Presbyterian Church. I picked up the phone and called him.

"Dick, I've just watched the Kathryn Kuhlman show. Are those healings real?"

"Yes, John, they're real," Dick answered. "But you'd have to attend one of these meetings at the Shrine Auditorium to believe it for yourself. Why do you ask?"

I hesitated, then spoke it out. "Dick, I've got something terribly wrong with me. I have cancer. I've already had it break out in three areas of my body and I'm afraid the next time it will kill me. I know I sound like I'm grasping at straws, but that's what a drowning man does."

"I'm going to have Miss Kuhlman call you personally," Dick said.

29

"Oh no," I objected. "I know she's far too busy to deal with a policeman in Houston. Just tell me where I can get her books."

"I'll send you the books," Dick said. "But I'm also going to ask her to call you, as a personal favor to me."

In less than a week she did call, at my home. "I feel like I know you already," she said, her voice sounding just like it did on TV. "We're putting your name on our prayer list, but don't put off coming to one of the meetings."

I did put it off. Sara and I both read her books and became avid watchers of the TV program. "Where have we been all our lives?" Sara asked. "I've never even heard of her before, yet she's world famous."

5. Desperate Flight

Like so many other Baptists, we simply didn't realize there was anything going on in the Kingdom of God outside the Southern Baptist Convention. Now our eyes were being opened, not only to other ministries and the gifts of the Spirit, but the power of God to heal. Could this be for me, too?

In February I knew my time was running out. Sara and the children encouraged me. "Daddy," Elizabeth said, "you go to California and we'll stay home and pray. We believe God will heal you."

I looked at Sara Ann. Her eyes were

moist as she nodded and said, "I believe He's going to heal you, too."

On Friday, February 19, I flew from Houston to Los Angeles. Old friends in Los Angeles loaned me their car and I found a motel in Santa Monica. But as a policeman and as a Baptist, I wanted to size up Miss Kuhlman before I attended the meeting on Sunday.

I learned she usually flew in from Pittsburgh the day before the service at the Shrine. I also checked around, using my knowledge as a policeman, and found out where she stayed. As a trained investigator, this was all the information I needed.

Early the next morning I was at her hotel. Being a policeman it was easy to get acquainted with the security officers and pump them for information. Before long they had told me what time Miss Kuhlman usually arrived.

I took a seat in the lobby and waited. An hour later the door opened and she walked in, looking exactly as I had pictured her. I knew I was brazen, but I intercepted her on the way to the elevator. "Miss Kuhlman," I said, "I'm that police captain from Texas."

She broke into a wide grin and exclaimed, "Oh yes! You've come to be healed."

We chatted for a few moments and I said, "Miss Kuhlman, I'm a born-again believer in Jesus Christ. I know I don't have to be healed to be a believer, because I'm already a believer. But you speak of something in your books that I want as much as I want physical healing."

"What is that?" she said, her eyes searching my face.

"I want to be filled with the Holy Spirit," I said.

"Oh," she smiled softly, "I promise you that you can have that."

"Well, even though I'm mighty sick, I'm still strong enough to get to the auditorium and get in line. I've read your books and know the plan for the services. I'll be over bright and early in the morning to get a good seat." I started to excuse myself and turn away.

"Wait!" she said. "I've got a feeling

33

about this and I have to be obedient to the Holy Spirit. You meet us here in the morning and we'll drive over together. You can follow us in your car."

I hesitated. "Miss Kuhlman, I've been a policeman so long, and I've cut so many corners to get into places; this time I don't want to do anything that might hinder my healing. I'll just go and stand in line with the others."

Miss Kuhlman's face bristled and her eyes began to glitter. "Now let me tell you something," she said with deliberation. "God is not going to heal you because you're good. He's not going to heal you because you're a police captain. He's certainly not going to heal you because of the way you get into that meeting."

She had to say no more. The next morning I followed her from her hotel to the Shrine Auditorium. We arrived at 9:35 a.m. Although the meeting wouldn't start until 1:00 p.m., the sidewalks in front of the huge auditorium were already packed with several thousand waiting people.

6. A Bathtub Full of Love

We went in through the stage entrance and Miss Kuhlman said, "Now, you just feel free to roam about this place until you see me meet with the ushers. When I meet with them, I want you with me."

I agreed and wandered off through the vast auditorium. The ushers, hundreds of them who had driven for many miles to volunteer their time, were busy setting up chairs for the 500-voice choir, roping off the section for the wheelchairs, seating those who had come on chartered busses, and preparing the room for what was about to take place. Even as I walked through the auditorium I could almost taste the expectancy. It was like electricity. Everybody was whispering in hushed tones, like the Holy Spirit was already present. How unlike my experiences in church services. I was feeling it too and suddenly I was no longer a policeman, no longer a Southern Baptist deacon. I was just a man filled with cancer, needing a miracle to live. I knew, if one was ever going to happen, this was the place.

One of the men introduced himself as Walter Bennett. Immediately I recognized his name. I had read his testimony in *God Can Do It Again*. His wife had been healed of a horrible disease. He took me around to the stage door where Naurine, his wife, was standing guard. Just seeing her in such radiant health, and knowing that she had been dying, gave me new hope and faith. I felt as if I wanted to cry.

"John," Walter said, "we have something in common. You are a Baptist deacon and I was a Baptist deacon too. Let's go have a cup of coffee."

We slipped out the side door and found

a nearby cafe. "There's a chance, after you're healed," Walter said, "that your fellow Baptists might not want to have anything to do with you." He grinned knowingly.

He spoke with such faith, as if he knew I was going to be healed. "I don't care what anyone thinks about me if I'm healed," I said, "just as long as God touches my body."

Walter smiled. I felt such love for this new friend. "Well, one thing we can be sure of," he said softly. "God hasn't brought you all this way for nothing. You're going to return to Houston a new man."

Having this fellow Baptist deacon speak with such faith filled me with excitement. I could hardly wait until the meeting started.

Back in the auditorium Miss Kuhlman was meeting with the ushers for last minute instructions before the doors opened. I joined them on stage.

"We have with us today a man who is a captain with the police force in Houston," she said. "He has cancer throughout his body and I'm going to pray for

37

him at this time. I want each of you
men to bow in prayer as I petition the
Lord in his behalf."

I realized this was something special.
I knew, from reading her books, that her
ministry was simply reporting what God
was doing as the great miracle services
got underway—and that she had no par-
ticular gift of healing herself. She mo-
tioned for me to come forward and
stretched out her hands toward me.

Even though this was the moment I
had waited for, I hesitated. I remembered reading in her books that often
when she prayed for people they fell
down on the floor. I had thought that
falling was all right for a few Pentecos-
tals, but it wasn't for a Baptist—and
certainly not for a police captain. But I
had no choice. I stepped forward and
let her pray for me.

Bracing my feet in my best Judo stance,
I waited as she touched me and prayed
for my healing. Nothing happened, but
as I started to relax I heard her say,
"And fill him, blessed Jesus, with Thy
Holy Spirit."

I felt myself reel, and thought, *This*

can't be. I reaffirmed my footing, one foot behind the other, and I heard it the second time, "And fill him with Thy Holy Spirit."

It felt like someone had his hands on my shoulders and was pushing me to the floor. I couldn't resist and crumpled to the stage. I struggled to regain my feet just in time to hear her say it the third time, "Fill him with Thy Holy Spirit." And I was down again.

This time I remained down for several minutes, like I was soaking in a bathtub full of love. Someone helped me to my feet and I heard her say, "Now find yourself a seat. We are going to open this place and in just a few minutes every seat will be taken."

I should have listened, for moments later the doors were thrown open and the people came pouring down the aisles like lava down the sides of a volcano. I fought my way up the aisle, pausing to look at a whole section filled with people in wheelchairs. I couldn't get my eyes off their faces. Some of them were so young, yet so twisted. I wanted to cry again. "Oh, Lord, am I selfish want-

ing a healing when there are so many
people here, some of them so young?''

7. I Could Run a Mile

As I stood looking, I heard, maybe for the first time in all my life, God's inner voice saying, "There's no shortage in my storehouse."

With new strength I made my way to the back and slowly, painfully, climbed the stairs to a seat on the first row of the balcony.

There was still time before the meeting started. The huge choir had taken its place on the platform and was doing some last minute rehearsing. As usual, I spent my time sizing up the various people who were sitting around me.

I introduced myself to the man beside me. "I'm Dr. Townsend," he said.

"Are you a medical doctor?" I asked, astonished that medical doctors would attend a healing service.

"Yes, I am," he said, pulling out one of his business cards. "I come because I get a great blessing. I just like to see the mighty working power of God." Then he introduced me to his family. "I've brought my dad here from out of state," he said. "This is his first meeting."

Seated across the aisle was one of my favorite TV actors. "Well, how about that," I mused silently. "Doctors and movie stars way up here in the balcony. They haven't come to be recognized, just to be a part of the meeting." I was impressed.

The service started. A beautiful girl, a fashion model whose face I had often seen on the cover of Sara's women's magazines, shared a brief testimony of what Jesus Christ meant in her life. I had been in many evangelistic meetings, but this one was different. Maybe it was the sense of expectancy. Maybe it was the sense of awe. Whatever it was, this was different from any other meeting I had ever attended.

Miss Kuhlman was speaking from the platform. "You know, I have been asked to set this Sunday aside for young people, but people come from such great distances and I just don't have the heart to say, 'Young people only.' However, since there are so many young people here today, I must speak to them."

Her message was brief and geared to the youth. She talked about the love of God and then gave one of the most challenging invitations I'd ever heard. Now if there's anything that impresses a Baptist it's numbers and movement. And when I saw almost 1,000 young people leaving their seats to come forward and make decisions for Jesus Christ, I was impressed. I was equally impressed that unlike most revival meetings I had attended, there was no fanfare, no tear-jerking stories. Just a simple invitation from this tall woman who said, "Do you want to be born again?" The kids responded, many of them literally running down the aisles to accept that challenge.

She seemed to forget the time as she dealt with them on the stage, praying for many of them individually. Finally they filtered back to their seats, but the congregation was sensing something else. It was about to happen.

"Father," she was whispering, so low I could hardly hear it, "I believe in miracles. I believe that You're healing today like You were when Jesus Christ was here. You know the need of the people here, all over this huge auditorium. I pray that you will touch them. In the name of Jesus I ask it. Amen."

Then there was silence. I could feel my heart pounding in my chest. I became aware of each cell in my body and could almost feel the warfare taking place in the spiritual places as the forces of the Holy Spirit did battle against the forces of evil over my body. "Oh, God," I prayed, worshiping, "Oh, God."

Suddenly she was speaking again, her voice coming rapidly as she received knowledge of what was happening in the auditorium.

"There is a man in the upper balcony, on my extreme right, who has just been

44

healed of cancer. Stand up, sir, in the name of Jesus Christ and claim this healing."

I looked up. She was pointing to the opposite side of the balcony. It was phenomenal. I could only stare in amazement, yet I felt the excitement building inside of me. This was real. I knew it was real.

"Do not come to the platform unless you know God has healed you," she emphasized. I glanced around and saw the personal workers moving up and down the aisles. They were interviewing and quizzing people who thought they had been healed, making sure only those who were genuinely healed came forward to testify.

The healings she was reporting seemed to be mostly in the balcony. They moved across from the right to the left.

"Two people are being healed of eye problems."

"A woman is being healed right now of arthritis. Stand up and claim your healing."

"You are seated right in the middle of the balcony," Miss Kuhlman said.

45

"You came today to receive your hearing. God has restored it. Take your hearing aid off. You can hear perfectly."

I looked. A woman in her forties was standing to her feet, pulling hearing aids out of both ears. The doctor sitting next to me was weeping and saying, "Thank you, Jesus." One of the personal workers was standing behind her whispering. I thought the woman was going to shout as she threw up her hands, praising God. She could hear.

The healings were coming in my direction across the balcony. "Lord, don't let them play out," I prayed. Then I remembered what He had whispered to me on the floor below—"There is no shortage in God's storehouse."

Suddenly Miss Kuhlman was pointing at the left balcony, right where I was sitting. "You have come a long way for your healing for cancer," she said. "God has healed you. Stand up in the name of Jesus Christ and claim it."

It was so far from the stage to the balcony. She had no idea I was up there. But her long, slender finger was pointing in my direction.

One of the things I had learned as a Baptist was to operate on faith, not feeling. I said, "O Lord, of course I want to be healed. But how do I know this is for me?"

Instantly that same inner voice, the one I had heard downstairs when I was looking at the wheelchair people, said, "Stand up!"

I stood. Without a feeling of any kind, I simply stood in obedience and faith.

Then I felt it. It was like being baptized in liquid energy. I had never felt such strength flowing through my body. I felt like I could have taken the Houston phone directory and ripped it to shreds.

A woman approached me. "Have you been healed of something?"

"I have," I declared, wanting to leap and run all at the same time.

"How do you know?" she asked.

"I've never felt so gloriously well. I hardly had enough strength to get to this seat and now, ooooh, I feel so good." All the time I was stretching and bending, doing things I hadn't been able to do in more than a year. "I feel like I could run a mile," I said.

"Then run right on down to the stage and testify," she said.

I did. But on the way I began to wonder. "What if there's someone here from Houston? I'm going to bound up there on the stage and she's going to put her hands on me and I'm going to hit the floor. What will they think?"

But I didn't care.

8. "Prove Me Now"

Moments later I was standing beside Miss Kuhlman on the stage. She just walked over to me and said simply, "We thank you, blessed Father, for healing this body. Fill him with the Holy Ghost."

Bam! I was on the floor again. This time, because of the new healing energy surging through my body, I bounced right back to my feet. The next time she didn't even touch me. She just prayed in my direction and I heard her say, "Oh, the power . . ." And I was on the floor again.

I stayed there this time, luxuriating in

49

that tub of liquid love again. But even there, Satan attacked me. He came on like a roaring lion. "What makes you think you've been healed?"

Miss Kuhlman had already turned her attention to someone else. I rolled over and came up on my knees, my head in my hands, praying. "Oh, Father, give me the faith to accept what I sincerely believe you've given me."

Across the years I had taken numerous Baptist study courses. My mind had been thoroughly exposed to the Word of God, and in that moment a verse came to me, "Prove me now herewith, saith the Lord of hosts."

I thought of all those twisted bodies I had seen. "Father, let me see a visible sign so my faith will be made strong."

I opened my eyes and coming to the platform was a little girl about nine years old. I had never seen anyone so happy. She was running and skipping, barefooted. She danced all the way across the stage, right by Miss Kuhlman who reached out to catch her but missed. She turned and started back. Again Miss

Kuhlman reached for her but she danced out of reach. By that time the child's mother was on the platform. She was holding a pair of shoes with heavy steel braces.

Unable to catch the dancing, skipping child, Miss Kuhlman turned to the mother. "What do we have here?"

The mother was sobbing. "This is my little girl. She had infantile paralysis when she was a baby and has never walked without these braces. But look at her go now."

The huge congregation broke into a mighty roar of applause.

"How do you know God has healed her?" Miss Kuhlman asked.

"Oh, I felt the healing power of God going through her body," the mother almost shouted. "I took the braces off and she began to run."

Right behind her was another mother, holding a two-year-old child. "What's this?" Miss Kuhlman asked.

"God has just made my baby's foot whole," the mother said, her voice shaking so hard she was hard to understand.

51

Miss Kuhlman reached out and took the baby's foot in her hands. "Was this the foot?"

"Yes, yes it was," the mother blurted out.

"But I see no difference in this foot and the other."

"But look at this," the mother said, holding a built-up shoe. "This child was born with a club foot. There have been many operations. Had you been massaging her foot the way you are turning it now, she would have screamed in pain."

Miss Kuhlman said, "On the platform with me are a number of doctors. They know me. Is there a doctor in the audience who doesn't know me and doesn't know these children, and would you come up and examine them?"

A man stood up.

"Are you a practicing physician, sir?" she asked.

"I am," he said.

"Where do you practice?"

"St. Luke's Hospital here in Los Angeles," he said.

52

"Would you please come up and examine these children?"

The doctor came to the platform. "The first thing I say is that this little girl, running and jumping on these toothpick legs, is a miracle. It's a miracle she can even stand on them, much less jump with joy." Then he took the infant's feet and held them together. "Miss Kuhlman," he said seriously, "I can see no difference in this child's two feet. I think this mother can throw away the therapeutic shoe."

I needed no more proof. I staggered back stage, found a coin telephone, and called Sara in Houston. The line was busy. I asked the operator to break in.

"I can't do that unless it is a matter of life and death," she said.

"That's exactly what it is, operator," I said. "And you can listen in if you want to."

9. Full of Color and Life

Suddenly Sara was on the phone. I tried to talk but all I could do was sob. I've never cried so hard in all my life, holding the phone and standing back stage at the Shrine Auditorium. Sara kept saying, "John, John, have you been healed?"

I finally got the message through. I was healed. Then she began to cry. I hoped the operator was listening. The call was about life, not death.

I made my way back to the edge of the stage and watched. Five Catholic priests, one of them a Monsignor, were sitting on the front row of stage chairs. The Monsignor was on the edge of his chair, drinking it all in. As Miss Kuhlman passed him she saw how intent he was. "Wouldn't you like this?" she asked.

He knew exactly what she was talking about because he stood to his feet, his robes flowing, and said, "Yes."

She put her hands on him and said, "Fill him with the Holy Ghost." Down he went. She turned to the other priests and said, "Come on." Each of them had the same falling experience.

Hippies being saved. Catholic priests being filled with the Holy Ghost. Twisted limbs straightened. My own cancer healed. I left early and drove back to the motel. It was more than I could comprehend.

In the motel I did all kinds of exercises —sit-ups, push-ups, things I hadn't been able to do in more than a year. And I did them with ease. Even without a medical examination, I knew I was healed. All that night I kept waking up, not to take pain pills (for I stopped all medication that morning before going to the service), but to say out loud in the darkness, "Thank you, Jesus. Praise the Lord!"

Then came the reunion with Sara and the children. They were waiting at the Houston airport when I arrived. Forgetting the crowd of people getting off the plane with me, I rushed to them, hugging Sara so tightly I literally picked her off the floor. She gasped at my strength. Then I grabbed the boys, first Andrew then John, picking them up and holding them over my head. We were all talking at once.

"Your face, John," Sara kept saying. "It's full of color and life."

"I knew you would be healed," Elizabeth was saying. "I prayed for you every day at 9, 12, and 6."

"Us too, Daddy," little John piped up. "Us little guys been praying too. We knew God would heal you."

It was too much, and this veteran police captain stood in the middle of the Houston airport and cried.

10. He Kept Repeating, "Remarkable!"

Shortly afterwards I returned for a physical examination. I made an appointment with two doctors from the M.D. Anderson Institute on the same day.

The first doctor to see me was the one who had performed the surgery. I carried her a copy of Miss Kuhlman's book, *I Believe in Miracles*. She glanced at the book, listened as I told her my story, and then looked at me like I was crazy.

"Let me tell you something," she said. "The only miracle that has happened to you is a medical miracle. That's all.

The only thing that's keeping you alive is your medication. You quit taking it and see how long you'll live.''

I smiled. "Well, I haven't had any medication since the 20th of February, more than a month ago.''

She was shocked and angry. "You've done a very foolish thing, Mr. LeVrier,'' she snapped. "It won't be long before that cancer breaks out someplace else and you'll be done.''

Such a strange attitude, I thought, for a scientist.

I left and went to Dr. Lowell Miller's office, chief of the Department of Radiation Therapy at Hermann Hospital. I hoped his reaction would be more positive, but after the last encounter I was determined not to tell him a thing about the miracle. He could just find out for himself.

His nurse asked me to go in the dressing room and prepare for a physical examination. She gave me one of those funny little white robes to put on, the kind that covers almost nothing in the front and is wide open in the back. I slipped off my pants to get dressed, and then noticed a strange thing. Like many long-time policemen, I had developed a good case of varicose veins in my legs. In fact, they had been so bad I wouldn't wear Bermuda shorts in public, for I was ashamed of the knots on my legs. Of course, when you're dying of cancer you don't worry about varicose veins, but in the bright light of the examination room I looked at my legs for the first time since returning from Los Angeles. Not only had the Lord healed me of cancer, He had healed the varicose veins also! My legs were as smooth as a young teenager's. By the time Dr. Miller came into the room I was bubbling over with praise.

Unaccustomed to seeing his cancer patients in such a joyful spirit, Dr. Miller stepped back. "My, what in the world has happened to you?"

That was all I needed to launch into the whole story of how Jesus Christ had healed my cancer.

"Now look," Dr. Miller said. "I'm a Christian too, but God has given us enough sense to look after ourselves."

"You'll get no argument from me on

61

that," I said gleefully. "That's the reason I'm here to be examined. I'll submit to any exam you want to give. But I'm telling you, you won't find anything wrong."

"Okay, let's go," the doctor said. And what followed was the most thorough physical examination I had ever had.

When he finished he said, "You know, I wish my prostate felt as good as yours." Then he went down my spine, beating on me, vertabrae by vertabrae. "Remarkable," he kept repeating. "Remarkable."

He sent me to X-ray and then said, "I'll call you in a day or so after I've compared these pictures with your old ones. But from all indications you've been healed."

Three days later the phone on my desk of the second floor office in the Houston Police Department rang. My secretary said it was Dr. Miller.

"Captain," he said, "I have good news. I can find absolutely no trace of cancer. Now, I want to ask you one other question. Do you ever bring talks?"

"You mean about my police work?" I said.

"No," he said, "not about police work. I want you to come out to my church and tell the people what God has done for you."

That opened the door, and I've been going ever since, all over the nation, telling hopeless people about the God who has no shortage in His storehouse of miracles.

Picture on the next two pages of Shrine Auditorium in Los Angeles, California.

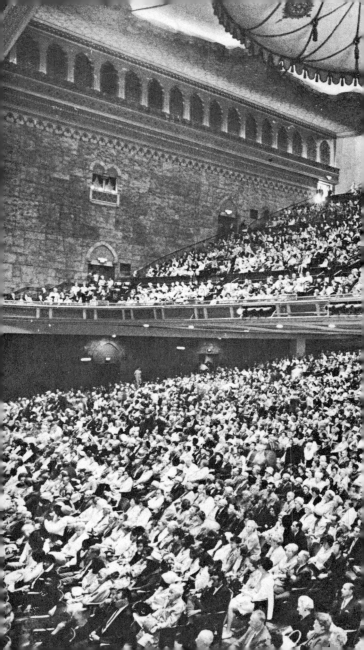

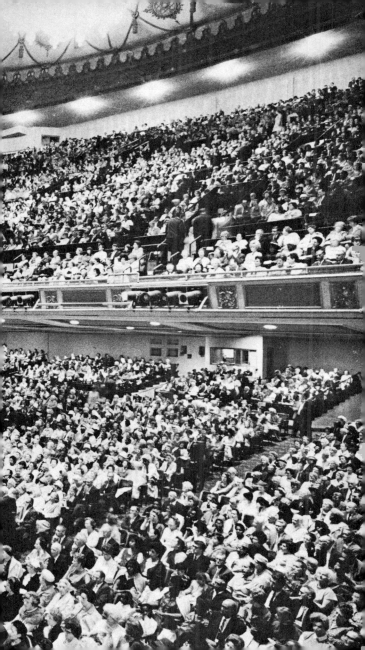

11. What Is the Key?

A *little* knowledge and an over-abundance of zeal always tends to be harmful. In the area involving religious truths, it can be disastrous.

Not long ago, a well-meaning person painted my portrait in oils. To the artist it was a masterpiece, but our radio announcer, who happened to be in the office as I was unwrapping the picture, took one look and in his quiet way commented, "An over-abundance of good intentions, but no talent!"

Often I am prone to react in exactly the same way to those who have so *much*

From the book, *I Believe in Miracles* by Kathryn Kuhlman, copyright © 1962 by Prentice-Hall, Inc. Published by Prentice-Hall, Inc., Englewood Cliffs, New Jersey.

to say about faith, those who profess to be authorities on the subject, who claim to have all the answers regarding faith healing, even to the point of judging those who fail to receive healing from the giving Hand of God.

In the early part of my ministry, I was greatly disturbed over much that I observed occurring in the field of Divine Healing. I was confused by many of the "methods" I saw employed, and disgusted with the unwise "performances" I witnessed—none of which I could associate in any way with either the action of the Holy Spirit or, indeed, the very nature of God.

Too often I had seen pathetically sick people dragging their tired, weakened bodies home from a healing service, having been told that they were not healed simply because of their own lack of faith. My heart ached for these people, as I knew how they struggled, day after day, trying desperately to obtain *more* faith, taking out that which they had, and trying to analyze it, in a hopeless effort to discover its deficiency which was presumably keeping them from the evitability of their defeat, because they were unwittingly looking at themselves, rather than to God.

But what *was* the answer? Again and again I was to ask myself the question: why were some healed and others not? Was there no balm in Gilead?

Was faith something that one could manufacture, or work up in oneself? Was it something that could be obtained through one's own goodness or moral status? Was it something that could be procured in exchange for serving the Lord, or through benevolence? I knew God could not lie, for He had promised; I knew in my own heart that there *was* healing, for I had seen the evidence from those who had been healed. It was real, and it was genuine, but *what was the key?*

I could not see the Hand of God in man's superfluity of zeal and I saw the harm that was being done in attributing everything to "lack of faith" on the part of the individual who had not received his healing. Inside myself, I was crushed: my heart told me that God could do anything; my mind told me that through

69

ignorance and lack of spiritual knowledge, there were those who were bring-
ing a reproach on something that was
sacred and wonderful and accessible
to all. No preacher had to tell me that
the Power of God was real and that God
knew no such thing as a MIRACLE as
such, for I was assured of these facts
as I read the Word of God. The Word
was there, the promise had been given:
there was surely no changing of God's
Mind, and certainly no cancelling of the
promises!

I think that no one has ever wanted
Truth more avidly than I—nor sought
it harder.

I remember well the evening when I
walked from under a big tent where a
Divine Healing service was being con-
ducted. The looks of despair and disap-
pointment on the faces I had seen, when
told that only their lack of faith was
keeping them from God, were to haunt
me for weeks.

Was this, then, the God of all mercy
and great compassion? I remember that
night how, with tears streaming down
my face, I looked up and cried: "They

have taken away my Lord and I know not where they have laid Him!'' And I remember going to my room and sobbing out my heart to God—praying for light on the Truth.

Fortunately I had learned a valuable spiritual lesson early in my ministry—one which was to come to my aid now: I had learned that the only way to get the truth is to come in sincerity and absolute honesty of heart and mind, and let the Lord Himself give one the blessed revelations of His Word, and *through* the Word, make His Presence real and His Truth known.

At no time in my search did I profess to wear the robe of infallibility. I did not seek as a dogmatist, nor as one with a closed mind, but only as one who was daily learning, willing to be guided by the Holy Spirit, and longing to be taught of the Father—as one who was hungry for deeper spiritual knowledge, not from man but from *God*.

I waited expectantly for the answer, and it came.

One night during a series of services that I was conducting, a very fine Christian lady arose from where she was sitting in the audience and said, "Please—before you begin your sermon, may I give a word of testimony regarding something that happened last evening while you were preaching?"

I nodded, and quickly recalled what I had said the night before. There had not been anything unusual about the sermon: it had been a very simple message regarding the Person of the Holy Spirit. I clearly recalled the sum and substance of the message:

God the Father is seated on His Throne, and is the Giver of every good and perfect gift. At His right Hand is His Son, through Whom we receive salvation and healing for our bodies, and in Whom every need of our lives is met. The Holy Spirit is the only member of the Trinity Who is here on earth and working in conjunction with the Father and the Son. He is here to do anything and everything for us that Jesus would do, were He here in Person.

I listened now, as the little woman spoke:

"As you were preaching on the Holy

Ghost," she said, "telling us that in Him lay the Resurrection power, I felt the Power of God flow through my body. Although not a word had been spoken regarding the healing of the sick, I knew instantly and definitely that my body had been healed. So sure was I of this that I went to the doctor today and had my healing verified."

The Holy Spirit, then, was the answer: an answer so profound that no human being can fathom the full extent of its depths and power, and yet so simple that most folk miss it!

I understood that night why there was no need for a healing line; no healing virtue in a card or a personality; no necessity for wild exhortations "to have faith."

That was the beginning of this healing ministry which God has given to me; strange to some because of the fact that hundreds have been healed just sitting quietly in the audience, without any demonstration whatsoever, and even without admonition. This is because the Presence of the Holy Spirit has been in such abundance that by His Presence alone

73

sick bodies are healed, even as people wait on the outside of the building for the doors to open.

Many have been the times when I have felt like taking the shoes off my feet, knowing that the ground on which I stood was Holy Ground. Many are the times when the Power of the Holy Ghost is so present in my own body that I have to struggle to remain on my feet. Many are the times when His Very Presence healed sick bodies before my eyes; my mind is so surrendered to the Spirit that I know the exact body being healed: the sickness, the affliction, and in some instances, the very sin in their lives. And yet I could not pretend to tell you *why* or *how!*

From the beginning, as now, I was wholly sure of two things: first, that I had nothing to do with what was happening, and second, I *knew* that it was the supernatural power of Almighty God. I have been satisfied to leave the why and the how to Him, for if I knew the answers to those two questions, then I would be God!

In the light of God's great love, tenderness and compassion, the Holy Spirit revealed to me my worthlessness and help-lessness of self. His greatness was over-whelming; I was only a sinner, saved by the Grace of God. The Power was His and the Glory, and this Glory, *His* Glory, He will not share with any human being.

If you can once grasp the concept of the Holy Trinity, many things which may once have puzzled you become clear. The Three Persons of the Trinity, God the Father, God the Son, and God the Holy Ghost are a Unity. They are co-existent—infinite and eternal. All Three were equally active in the work of creation, and are equally active and indispensable in the work of Redemption. But although the Three work together as One, each has at the same time His own distinctive function.

God the Father planned and purposed the creation and the redemption of man, and is in our vernacular, the Big Boss. God the Son provided and purchased at Calvary what the Father had planned in eternity. He made possible the realiza-tion of God's eternal plan. All that we receive from the Father *must* come through Jesus Christ the Son, and that

is why at the heart of our faith is a
Person—the very Son of the very God.
When we pray, we come before the Father's Throne in Jesus' Name. We cannot
obtain an audience with the Father, except as we come to Him in the Name
of His Son.

But the Holy Spirit is the *power* of the
Trinity. It was *His* power which raised
Jesus from the dead. It is the *same* Resurrection power that flows through our
physical bodies today, healing and
sanctifying.

In short, when we pray in the Name
of Jesus, the Father looks down through
the complete perfection, the utter holiness, the absolute righteousness of His
only Begotten Son, knowing that by Him,
the price was paid in full for man's redemption, and *in* Him lies the answer
to every need.

God honors the redemptive work of
His Son by giving to us through Him
the desire of our hearts. Thus, while it
is the Resurrection power of the Holy
Spirit which performs the actual healing
of the physical body, Jesus made it perfectly clear that we are to look to Him,

the Son, in faith, for He is the One who has made all these things possible.

Faith

Volumes have been written and volumes more have been spoken regarding this indefinable something called *faith*, and yet in the final analysis we actually know so little of the subject.

Faith is that quality or power by which the things desired become the things possessed. This is the nearest to a definition of faith attempted by the inspired Word of God.

You cannot weigh it or confine it to a container: it is not something that you can take out and look at and analyze: you cannot definitely put your finger on it and positively say, "This is it." To explain it precisely and succinctly is almost like trying to define energy in one comprehensive statement. In the realm of physics we are told that the atom is a world within itself, and that the potential energy contained within this tiny world is such that it bewilders the mind of the average person. Attempt to define it, and you will run into difficulties. And so it is with faith in the realm of the spirit. But although it is not easy to define exactly what faith *is*, we know what it is *not*.

One of the most common errors we make in this regard is to confuse faith with presumption. We must be constantly alert to the danger of mistaking one for the other, for there is a vast difference between the two.

There is a pebble on the beach, for example, but the beach is more than the pebble. When the pebble asserts that it is the beach, then we say to it: "You are assuming too much."

There are many who mix the ingredients of their own mental attitude with a little confidence, a pinch of trust and a generous handful of religious egotism. They proceed to add some belief, along with many other ingredients, and mixing it in a spiritual apothecary's crucible, they label the total result *faith*. Actually, the consequence of this heterogeneous mixture is more likely to be presumption than faith.

Faith is more than belief; it is more

than confidence; it is more than trust, and above all, it is never boastful. If it is pure faith, Holy Ghost faith, it will never work contrary to the Word of God, and neither will it work contrary to His wisdom and will.

There have been times when I have felt faith so permeate every part of my being that I have dared to say and do things which, had I leaned to my own understanding or reason, I would never have done it. Yet it flowed through every word and act with such irresistible power that I literally stood in wonder at the mighty works of the Lord. One thing I know: in you and in me apart from God, there are *no* ingredients and *no* qualities which, however mixed or combined, will create even so much as a mustard seed of Bible faith.

Let us just reason together in a very simple understanding way: if I wanted to cross a lake, and there were no means of getting across except by boat, the sensible thing for me to do would be to secure a boat. It would be most foolish for me to seek the other side of the lake, when I needed to seek the proper conveyance to get there. Get the boat and it will take you there.

Now, where do we get the faith that will take us across the lake? The answer to this question is positive and sure!

Faith is a gift of God or a fruit of the Spirit, and whether it be gift or fruit, the source and the origin of faith remain the same. It comes from God and is a gift of God.

If faith is powerless, it is not faith. You cannot have faith without results any more than you can have motion without movement. The thing we sometimes call faith is only trust, but although we trust in the Lord, it is *faith* which has action and power.

A man might well trust the Lord and His promise that some day he would be saved and that some day he would accept Christ in the forgiveness of his sins: he might well trust the Lord sufficiently to believe that God had the ability to forgive his sins. But it is only if this man possesses an active, power-filled *faith* for salvation that he can be "born again."

80

"By grace are ye saved, through faith; and that not of yourselves; it is the gift of God."

Grace and faith are so closely related that you cannot separate one from the other. The wonder of it all is the fact that many times faith is imparted when we feel the least deserving. But faith is not the product of merit, for no human being *deserves* salvation, and no person living merits the smallest of God's blessings: that is why the two, grace and faith, are so closely related.

The faith imparted to the sinner for salvation is solely the result of God's mercy and grace. It is a gift. The faith that is imparted to the individual for the healing of his physical body is again only the result of God's mercy—the overflow of His great compassion and grace. It is a gift. You do not pray for faith; you seek the Lord, and faith will come.

The disciples and the Master were on the waters of Galilee. It was a beautiful day; the lake was calm and serene, and there was scarcely a cloud in the sky—when suddenly, a terrific storm arose! The poor disciples were terror-stricken. The wind was blowing in all its fury, the little boat was about to capsize, and they were certain that their very lives were at stake.

Finally in desperation they awakened the sleeping Christ. Calmly, without perturbation, He asked just one question: "Where is your faith?" (Luke 8: 25).

Where was it? Had they left it on shore before entering the boat? Had it dropped to the depth of the sea on which their little boat was sailing? Had it fled on the shoulders of the storm?

Their faith had been resting in the stern of the boat!

Their faith was with them all the time. It had never left them for one second. *He* was their faith; but the mistake they had made was in forgetting the fact of His Presence while discerning the fact of the storm! That is exactly what Jesus meant when He said, "Without me ye can do nothing." *He*, then, is your faith.

We become defeated when we fasten our eyes on circumstances, our own problems, our weaknesses, our physical illnesses. The surest way to be defeated is to focus our mind on ourselves. The storm will capsize our little boat, of that we can be sure, and yet, the fact remains that our faith for victory was nearer to us than our hands or feet.

No person need ever be defeated on a single score; no person needs to lack faith. Look up, as Carey Reams did, and see Jesus! He is your faith, He is our faith. It is not faith that you must seek, *but Jesus*.

The Giver of every good and perfect gift is the Author and Finisher of our faith!

I Believe

that the Holy Bible is the Word of the Living God; that it is the supernaturally inspired Word; that it was written by holy men of old as they were moved and inspired by the Holy Ghost; that it is the only true ground of Christian unity and fellowship. That it is the eternal tribunal by whose standards all men and nations shall be judged.

I believe in the Trinity: Father, Son and Holy Ghost, as three separate individuals; equal in every Divine perfection.

I believe in God the Father Almighty, Creator of heaven and earth, Whose glory is so exceeding bright that mortal man cannot look upon His face and live. His nature so transcends human standards of comparison that a definition is impossible. If a demonstration of God's existence were possible, He would be too limited to fill the office of Supreme Being and Ruler of the Universe. Faith begins where reason and logic end!

I believe that Jesus Christ is the very Son of the Living God, co-existent and co-eternal with the Father, who was conceived by the Holy Ghost and born of the Virgin Mary, taking upon Himself the form of man, and by the shedding of His blood, made atonement for fallen man.

Just as prophecy is the unanswerable argument in the realm of Eternal Evidence, so the Person of Jesus Christ is the unanswerable argument in the realm of Internal Evidence. Not only does His entire life fulfill perfectly the Old Testament prophecies, but His Person, towering as it does above every other, is beyond explanation only as we admit Him to be Very God as well as Very Man.

The miraculous life of Christ is an unanswerable argument for His miraculous birth!

I believe the Holy Spirit is a Person, and a Divine Person, and not just a Divine influence. The marks of personality are knowledge, feeling and will, and any being who knows, thinks, feels and wills, is a person whether he has a body or not. All the distinctive marks or characteristics of personality are ascribed to the Holy Spirit in the Word.

As a member of the eternal Trinity, the Holy Ghost has aided in the creation of the earth and its forms of life. He was present at the creation of man. Hence the words: "Let *us* make man." It was foreordained from before the foundation of the world that the Holy Ghost should be dominant and controlling in the Church.

I believe that by voluntary disobedience and transgression man fell from innocence and purity to the depths of sin and iniquity.

Because of man's fallen state, judgments had to be met, law had to be satisfied, penalties had to be paid; all of these things the holiness of God required.

Jesus Christ the Son, through the Holy Ghost, offered Himself to God the Father as a propitiation for sin; that is why Christ is referred to as "The lamb slain from the foundation of the world."

The blood of Christ is so effective that it not only cleanses from all sin, but one day the effect of that blood shed in Jerusalem nineteen hundred years ago will remove the curse of sin from the earth.

His sinless blood is a sufficient atonement for our sin!

I believe in salvation as a *definite* experience—an experience through which the individual is no longer under the bondage of sin, but "is passed from death unto life," transformed by the Power of the Spirit. Quite literally "a new creature in Christ Jesus."

By simple faith, belief in God's Son,

and acceptance of Him as Divine Saviour, the guilty sinner is made righteous.

I believe in that "called out" body of believers, composed of Jew and Gentile, and individuals from every kindred, people, tribe and nation, originating at Pentecost, and known as "The Body of Christ."

I believe that the only way Jesus, Who is now at the right hand of God, as Great High Priest, can manifest Himself to the world is through His Body, the Church.

I believe that this Body, comprised of those who have been washed in the shed blood of the Son of God, is to be the Bride of Christ and will reign with Him in His millennial glory.

I believe in miracles!

Other books
you may want to read . . .

I'M NOT MAD AT GOD
by David Wilkerson
In this unique book David Wilkerson opens up his heart to tell us of the inner conflicts and victories. Its message has a keen cutting edge and a practicality not often found in books with a devotional flavor. Over 100,000 copies sold in hard cover. 75¢

AFTER ITS KIND
by Byron C. Nelson
A clear and thorough discussion of the theory of evolution. It is not merely critical, it is constructive. It meets and refutes the evolutionist on his own ground and gives the best authorities for every position taken. $1.95

THE DELUGE STORY IN STONE
by Byron C. Nelson
This book, along with AFTER ITS KIND, is a classic in the area of defending a creationist point of view and is usually quoted by contemporary writers on the subject. $1.95

RULED BY THE SPIRIT
by Basilea Schlink

A very practical book on how to live the Spirit-filled life. Several testimonies by Basilea Schlink's associates are included showing how one may enter into this Spirit-filled life. 95¢

SPEAKING IN TONGUES
by Larry Christenson

Corrie ten Boom says in the foreword: "I know that God will use this book to open the eyes of many of his children to the privilege of living in a time when God is pouring out his blessings of the gifts and fruit of the Spirit on different churches." 95¢

UNION AND COMMUNION
by J. Hudson Taylor

A study of the Song of Solomon in which the author unfolds in simplest language the deep truths of the believer's personal union with the Lord. 75¢

LIKE A DOVE DESCENDING
by Ian Macpherson

Here's a clear, revealing exposition of the nature and work of the Holy Spirit. It is not primarily a theological discourse, but rather a practical illustration of what the Holy Spirit has come to accomplish in the life of every child of God. $1.00

STARS, SIGNS, AND SALVATION IN THE AGE OF AQUARIUS
by James Bjornstad and Shildes Johnson

Astrology—where did it all begin? Is astrology really valid? Is it compatible with Judaism and Christianity? Read and consider the authors' sometimes unsettling but always logical conclusions. 95¢

WHEN GOD CALLS
by Basilea Schlink
Here's a book that thousands of Basilea Schlink readers have been waiting for—her personal autobiography. Her early years in Hitler's Germany and her founding of the Evangelical Sisterhood of Mary make fascinating reading for anyone. $1.25

AS HE WALKED
by Ernst I. Dahle
This book shows how a normal human being who is naturally self-loving, self-centered, and self-seeking can become equally naturally God-loving and other-loving. 75¢

MY ALL FOR HIM
by Basilea Schlink
Meditations on how to live for Christ and why this "way" brings true happiness. $1.25

WHY JESUS
by F. J. Huegel
A very simple yet profound book showing why Jesus is the one person that everyone will someday have to face, and either accept or reject. $1.00

PRAYING HYDE
by Francis McGaw
John Hyde stands out as a testimony to what God can do in and through the life of one who is willing to pray, believe, and *act*. 75¢

Purchase these books at your **local bookstore**. If your local bookstore does not have these books, you may order from **Bethany Fellowship, Inc.,** 6820 Auto Club Road, Minneapolis, Minnesota 55438. Enclose payment with your order, plus 10¢ per book for postage.